Positive Healer

Nery Román

ISBN-13:
978-1727897548

ISBN-10:
1727897544

Love yourself and don't be afraid to express who you are ... Be a proud Latino!

Your positive action joint with positive thinking causes success... Together Latinos

Live life to the maximum and concentrate on the positive... Latin Power

Stay positive and happy... Latinos

Every day begins with a positive attitude and wanting to improve...
Latino

"He begins to live, counting each day separately, as an independent life."

Break the routine and you'll get what you want in life. Latino

The only way to avoid failure is to keep trying anything.

Don't be afraid to fail... that's how you achieve it.

Besides, it's just really a flop if you stop trying.

Let's not be jealous. Jealousy is a destructive emotion... Latino

People who are not happy are filled with an emotional emptiness through negative emotions. Be positive...
Latino

It's about believing in you Latino, when no one does...

Long live freedom of speech. Latin

Take the first step, fear will not follow… Latin

Overcome the fear of failure by visualizing the worst case. Latino

When we are thinking about fear, negativity, concern, doubt, criticism, judgment, anger, frustration, anxiety, negativity and others, we are not focused on what we want.

"How do you live life to the fullest?"

Latino?

What have you done today to live life to the maximum Latino?

Use your failures to learn from them and be stronger, Latino...

Be creative, without being afraid of what others say...

When we are focused on what we do not want, everything we see, our ideas and decisions are based on what we do not want.
Latino

When we know what we want, we give ourselves the ability to imagine new possibilities and generate ideas on how to be and what to do or say at every moment. We make it a reality. Latino...

Powerful effect = survive and prosper... Latino

When faced with the reality of losing, immigration, we can think about what is important "our families," Latino...

When all members of your family are happy, this contributes to your individual success and to your Latino Family...

The investment we make now returns to us with twice as much blessing.

We have a great task because we are Latinos...

Be a better person and you will be able to achieve greatness and prosper. Latinos...

Keep a diary of gratitude... Latinos.

Count your Latino blessings....

Be happy

Nery Román